The Diagnosis Of Sexual Ambiguities

Introduction

The reader in the topics of Gender Identity Disorder and homosexuality is going to encounter many tangled terms that might be mistaken by the inexpert for synonyms, but after a careful and close study of them, a real difference will be found between them.

Gender Identity Disorder:

Gender Identity Disorder is divided into:

1. Transgender: which is a rare condition where the person feels that they belong to the opposite sex although they don't have genital deformation.
2. Intersex: it is a condition where the gender of the person can't be identified using the traditional ways due to a genetic, genital, or hormonal disorder and its treatment differs according to the condition.

People with Gender Identity Disorder are treated by a team that consists of a pediatric surgeon and a psychiatrist in the case of the young children. But in the case of the adults, they are treated by a team of a urologist surgeon, a gynecologist, and a psychiatrist.

And as for the paraphilia, it only needs the treatment of a psychiatrist as it is a disorder in only the sexual preferences and not in the sexual identity.

Homosexuality:
It is a sexual orientation that is identified by the sexual and emotional attraction toward the people of the same gender more than toward the other gender.

Homosexual behavior: it is the action of seeking sexual satisfaction through having sexual activities between people from the same gender. It is divided into being gay or lesbian according to the gender of the people involved.

The person who has homosexual orientation didn't necessarily have homosexual activities and who practiced it is not necessarily a homosexual.

And by looking at the statistics about the homosexuality without any regard to these differences, they will be found conflicted, but by considering these differences between the terms, the differences in the statistics will be understood.

For example, the homosexual people represent between 1 to 3% of the Us and Canada's population; although 20% of the Americans stated that they felt attraction to the same gender before but without practicing any homosexual activities. But when looking at the statistics about the homosexual activities, we will find that between 5-10% of the Americans had homosexual activities at least once, whereas only 1% of the Americans consider themselves homosexual.

Is it right that the homosexual people represent 10% of the society?

Many societies and organizations supporting the homosexual rights claim that they represent more than 10% of the society, but this is not true as many studies by the American CDC showed that they represent only 2% of the American society.

We will basically consider, in this focus, the problems posed in clinical practice by ambiguous sexual developments and how to solve them, the pathogenic considerations being mentioned only insofar as they are necessary for the comprehension, and thus to the treatment of abnormalities of sexual development. Let us insist from the outset on the absolute necessity of an early diagnosis, since any mistake in the sex attributed to a child is with catastrophic consequences on the somatic and psychological levels, because from around the age 3, the child becomes so fixed in his "psychological sex" that any "change of sex" becomes an extremely hazardous enterprise, if not impossible.

Definition

It must be understood under the name of "sexual ambiguity" or "Hermaphroditism" any case where there is a discrepancy between the criteria of the normal sexual determination. Therefore, and this is an important introductory remark, one may be led to make the diagnosis of "sexual ambiguity" or "hermaphroditism" in a child whose external genital aspect is obviously masculine or feminine, where the examination is being motivated by growth disorders or pubertal development.

The Criteria Of Sexual Determination

The study of the criteria of the sexual determination is the necessary preamble to study the various anomalies. The notions of embryology essential for the understanding of pathological cases will be recalled first.

1) **Genetic sex.** It is determined from fertilization by the chromosomal formula of the cell resulting from the union of the spermatozoon and the ovum. This formula is, as we know, either type XX, that is, female; or of the XY type, that is to say, male. Recent work has shown that the number of chromosomes in the human species is 46, 23 pairs including 44 autosomes and 2 sex heterochromosomes (XX or XY). But in some cases of sexual ambiguity, we could highlight, by the tissue culture technique an abnormal chromosomal formula (or 47 chromosomes instead of 46) which might explain later anomalies of gonadogenesis and sexual development. Of course, these are delicate techniques that are not yet applicable in clinical practice. On the other hand, one can easily determine the chromatin sex. Moor and Barr have shown that any cell of the body bearing its chromatin mark, male or female, making it sufficient to study a smear of the oral mucosa suitably colored to know whether the chromatin sex was masculine or feminine (we currently prefer the terms chromatin sex positive (female) or negative (masculine)). In the female sex,

2) more than 80% of the cells studied have a perinuclear chromatin mass, while in the male sex, the chromatin is disseminated into irregular grains (5% maximum cells with a chromatin clump). Although one can not assimilate chromatin and chromosome sex (or genetics), this is an essential examination that provides considerable services in the study of sexual ambiguities.

3) Gonadic Sex. It is defined by the presence of testes or ovaries. It is known that at the beginning of the intrauterine life, the genital crest first appears (around the 30th day). which will be colonized secondarily by the germinal cells. We distinguish then in this pro gonad or primitive gonad, identical in both sexes, a central or medullary zone and a peripheral or cortical zone. The male or female sexualization of the pro gonad occurs around the 45th day and seems dependent on the chromosome sex and "inductors" leading either to the development of the medulla, that is, the formation of a testicle or; the development of the cortex,: that is, the formation of an ovary. Clinically, gonadal sex can only be determined by exploratory laparotomy and biopsy for histological examination of both gonads. Gonadal sex, testes or ovaries, depends on the hormonal sex, that is, the secretion of androgens or estrogens that will be clinically appreciated by the determination of androgens (17 ketosteroids) and estrogens (Folliculin). Likewise depends on gonadal sex, Gametic Sex, that is to say the formation of spermatozoa or eggs.

4) Morphological Sex.
 It is divided into internal genital sex or gonophoric (in zoology, relating to the gonophore, polyp ensuring

reproduction in a colony of siphonophores), and external genital sex. The internal genital sex is characterized, in the female sex, by the presence of tubes, uterus, and vagina; while it is characterized in the male sex, by the epididymis and deferens. This differentiation is done by the development of Wolff's ducts in humans, and Muller's canals in women. The fundamental work of Jost showed that this differentiation is dependent on the secretion of the fetal gonad, specifically, the secretion of "virilizing hormones" (virilizing: which causes in the female the appearance of male secondary sexual characteristics.), by the fetal testis which is essential for the development of the genital tract in the male sense.

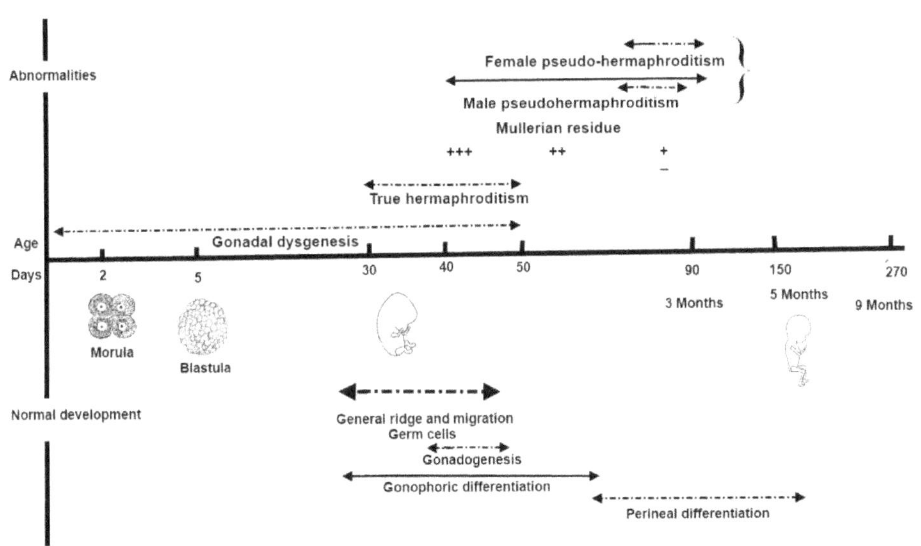

(picture 1) Chronology of successive stages of sexual differentiation and corresponding anomalies

In the absence - anatomical or functional - of the fetal testicle, the development of the genital tract will be in the feminine sense, even if the chromatin sex is masculine, and this, more or less, according to the more or less complete deficiency of the fetal testicle (notion of critical phases of Jost). The development of the genital tract according to the female type is therefore a passive phenomenon that will occur, of course, if the fetal gonads are ovaries; but if they are testicles not secreting, for some reason, or if the fetal gonads (testes or ovaries) have not developed or regressed, as we shall see, we have here the explanation of male Pseudohermaphroditism and some gonadal dysgenesis (picture 1).

In clinic, the determination of gonophoric sex will be made by the gynecological examination; by opacification, followed by the taking of X-rays, genitourinary tract (looking, especially a vaginal cavity); by laparoscopy or better by the exploratory laparotomy that allows only a complete assessment and necessary biopsies.

External genital sex, that is to say, the appearance of the external genital organs and the pinnate, feminine or masculine, which obviously determines the "sex of civil status". This differentiation is made from the uro-genital sinus of the fetus, with double sexual potentiality. In the male, the genital slit closes, the genital bulges give the scrotum, and the genital bud develops in penis, at the end of which opens the urethra penis. In the female, the urogenital sinus remains open (vulvar cleft), the genital bulges give the big lips, the genital bud increases to form the clitoris

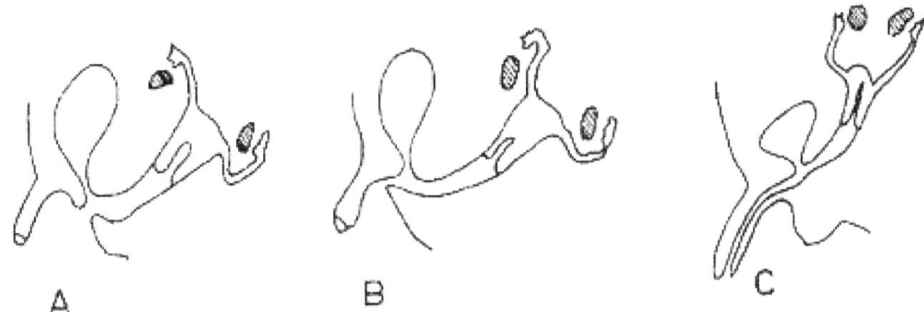

Anatomical disposition of female pseudo-hermaphrodisms by congenital adrenal hyperplasia (according to WILKINS, modified)

and the sinus is divided into ventral urethra and dorsal vagina. This differentiation is active in the male sex, that is to say requires the intervention of the fetal testicle, and passive in the female sex. It is important to emphasize that the urogenital sinus, unlike the gonophore, is sensitive not only to "androgens" of fetal origin, but also to hormones of maternal origin, that are secreted by the mother, or that are hormones that have been injected for therapeutic purposes. There will be shown here the explanation of many cases of female Pseudohermaphroditism.

In the clinic, the external genital sex is, of course, determined by the examination of the genitals and the perineum, but in case of ambiguous aspect, in no case should the morphological information be used to decide the sex to be attributed to the child, instead, the series of test that have just been mentioned must be implemented. In addition, let us insist on the need for a psychological assessment, whose importance is at least equal to the somatic balance sheet for the decisions to be made. Psychological problems, being common to the different types of anomalies, will be exposed at the end of this study.

Clinical Types of Sexual Determination Abnormalities

The sexual anomalies will be classified, not in a theoretical way, according to their pathogenesis, but in a clinical way, that is to say according to whether the external genital aspect is ambiguous or normal (male or female).

External Genital Aspect Ambiguity (Table 1)

If the external genital aspect is ambiguous, it is obviously for this anomaly that the pediatrician is consulted, too often late. Anyway, the malformation is obvious, the genital morphology is more or less similar to that of a boy or a girl. The genital bud can be described as "hypoplastic penis" as well as "hypertrophied clitoris". At the end, a blind mute depression, it is by removing the genital bulges of more or less "bursiform" appearance that we find either two orifices, a single orifice or urogenital sinus. All in all, this anatomical arrangement have often been considered as a "hypospadias vulvi form" and is treated, wrongly, later.

The first diagnosis that must be considered before such an aspect, is the one Congenital Adrenal Hyperplasia, which is the cause of many of the most frequent female pseudo-hermaphroditism (by definition the term, female pseudo-hermaphroditism refers to a subject with ambiguous external genital morphology;

whose chromatin sex is female and whose gonads are ovaries) and the only one of the pseudo-hermaphroditism which has a specific medical treatment (dexamethasone).

Genital Morphology: Ambiguous

Size	Age Bony	Clitoral hypertrophy	Pubic hair	Chromatinic sex	Opacification Genitourinary	Urinary Steroids	Gonads	Notice
Congenital adrenal hyperplasia								
↗	↗	+	+	♀	Vagina +	17 CS ↗ PG ↗	Ovary Laparotomy Useless	Very common
Female pseudo-hermaphroditism								
N	N	+	-	♀	Vagina +	N	Ovary	Relatively rare
Male Pseudohermaphrodism								
N	N	Penis + Or - aplastic	-	♂	Vagina ±	N	Testicles	Frequent
Hermaphroditism True								
N	N	±	-	♂ Or ♀	Vagina ±	N	Testicles + Ovary	Exceptional

1) **Female pseudo-hermaphroditism by congenital adrenal hyperplasia:**

Clinically, besides the genital malformation, the essential fact is the existence of signs of active hormonal stimulation, whereas other sexual ambiguities are only "scars" of the intrauterine life, with no signs of hormonal activity until the normal age of puberty. Therefore, local morphological examination will show not only a large genital bud (clitoral hypertrophy), but we also learn that it continues to increase gradually and is accompanied by a marked development of genital bulges (labia majora); especially that it has developed a pubic hair that increases regularly. At these signs of virilism, the general morphological examination makes it possible to add an advance of growth: the size is greater than normal, the highly developed muscle masses, often acne and axillary hair already exist. X-rays show a significant advance in bone age, often the sesamoid of the thumb is present.

Complementary examinations will be conducted according to the previously detailed plan: the first major fact is that the female chromatin sex proves that it is a "genetic daughter", virilized, and genito-urinary opacification draw a usually normal vagina. The decisive evidence of congenital adrenal hyperplasia is provided by hormonal assays that show a very high urinary excretion of 17 ketosteroids and an abnormal metabolite, the Prégnanetriol signature of the congenital metabolic abnormality at the origin of hyperplasia;

the 17 CSs and the pregnanetriol are brought back to normal levels for the chronological age by the administration of a suitable dose of dexamethasone, and it is there,-the diagnostic test is considered the beginning of the treatment.

TREATMENT: The specific treatment is in fact the corticotherapy aiming at curbing the hypersecretion pituitary ACTH. The most active pituitary blocker currently is dexamethasone. We will look for the minimum dose necessary and sufficient to maintain the urinary steroids at a normal rate (The usually required dose is of the order of 1 mg per day). This is a hormonal substitution therapy and must therefore be continued indefinitely. Thanks to the treatment - provided, of course, that it is undertaken early enough - puberty will occur at a normal age in the feminine sense (breasts, rulers) and fertility will be possible. Sometimes plastic surgery will be needed to enlarge the vulvar opening and reduce the size of the clitoris. A single anomaly is obviously irreversible: the advancement of bone age. So, if the treatment is undertaken only late, when the bone welds are already being completed, these big kids will become small adults.

But, sometimes, the diagnosis is not made before puberty and in the following observation, which is truly dramatic, the diagnosis was unknown until the age of 17! From birth, the external genital aspect makes you hesitate about sex: the child is declared as a girl and 15 days later as a boy; and it is like boy that he will be raised now. At the age of 5, appears and develops a pubic hairiness; from 8 years old, acne, finally the growth of stature, first fast, stops at two years old.

All these anomalies are not without worrying parents, but have told them that it is a hypospade to operate towards puberty. When we see the "young man", he is 17 years old and has an absolutely masculine general morphology, almost athletic, with a moderate statural delay. Pubic hair is stretched in a triangle across the pubic area and borders the genital cleft limited by a large labia appearance.

At the upper end thereof, the genital bud, 2 to 3 cm, presents the morphology of a clitoris, without an orifice at its end. The latter (uro-genital sinus) is carried back and down, and its opacification injects a well-developed genital cavity and even a trunk. The already obvious diagnosis will be confirmed by the female chromatin sex, the 17 CSs urinary at 220 mg 24 hours. This intelligent "boy" suffers from his small size and especially from his genital anomaly; he is afraid of not being able to found a home and to have a normal love. He is currently in love with a girl and her sexuality has always been oriented, without ambiguity, towards the female sex **(picture 2)**.

(picture 2) Opacification of the genitourinary tract: vaginal cavity, trunk

The problem therefore arises as follows: should we reveal the error and turn this boy into a girl, which would naturally be easy and very satisfactory from the somatic point of view, but without doubt catastrophic from the psychological point of view, or should we leave him as a boy, for the same reasons, so castrate and treat this clitoris as the penis of a hypospade. After long deliberation and agreement with the father of the child, it is this last solution which has been adopted, because one was in front of a masculine personality whose balance was acquired on the adult mode. (Even with the child being ovariectomized, it did not seem appropriate to give dexamethasone to partially curb the hypersecretion of androgens).

Such disasters must be avoided. Indeed if, in the infant the diagnosis can be for a certain time difficult because of the absence of hairiness and obvious advance in stature, genital ambiguity, absolutely imposes the study, from the first days of life, chromatin sex and urinary steroids that leave no doubt. Recall that in the neonatal period, the genital anomaly can be associated with a syndrome of adrenal insufficiency (uncontrollable vomiting, cardiovascular collapse) known as Debre-Fibiger syndrome which is a very serious prognosis despite the treatment with cortisone and deoxycorticosterone. Finally, a relatively rare form although of great theoretical interest, which should be cited where sexual ambiguity is associated with high blood pressure.

Pathogenesis:

We will quickly recall the diagram, now classic Eberlein and Bongiovanni. The fundamental disorder is the absence of a C**21** hydroxylase preventing the adrenal synthesis of the hydrocortisone. Due to this congenital metabolic abnormality, whose signature is the presence of pregnantriol in the urine, there is hypersecretion by the ACTH pituitary (normally inhibited by hydrocortisone) and, in return, hypersecretion by the adrenal cortico-steroids androgenic (hence high elimination of 17 CS) and progressive virilization. It will suffice to give a sufficient dose of hydrocortisone to curb the hypersecretion of ACTU and, in return, hypersecretion of adrenal androgens. In forms with high blood pressure, the deficient enzyme would be a $C11$-hydroxylase. In fact this diagram, if it remains true, does not explain all the cases, partial deficits are certainly possible and other abnormalities in the enzymatic chain of events seem likely.

2) Female pseudo-hermaphroditism without a congenital adrenal hyperplasia

The ambiguous external genital aspect, the female chromatin sex, and the presence of a vaginal cavity are common elements with the forms of hyperplasia. But two essential characters make it possible to differentiate them: clinically, there is no evidence of active hormonal stimulation (no statural or bone advance, no premature hair growth, and if clitoral hypertrophy exists, it does not progress: we are in the presence of a "scar" dating from intra-uterine life; and biologically, the hormonal assays (17 CS in particular) are normal for the chronological age of the child.

On the other hand, the diagnosis of true hermaphroditism, although extremely rare, can only be removed by exploratory laparotomy with a biopsy of both gonads - which in addition will allow a correct anatomical assessment (and therefore the evaluation of the subsequent functional possibilities).

Pathogeny:

If we conform to Jost's theories, we must admit (the chromatin sex being feminine, and the gonads having developed at the expense of the cortex of the primitive gonad to become normal ovaries) the partial virilization of the fetus at the beginning of the intrauterine life. This virilization being an active phenomenon, we must assume the intervention of a "virilizing substance", of endogenous origin or exogenous. If we admit the endogenous origin, two sources are possible; maternal or fetal. Apart from the cases, a virilizing tumor (ovarian arrhenoblastoma,) which is of course exceptional, where the mother was a carrier, during pregnancy, the maternal or fetal placenta or adrenal gland may constitute this abnormal and transient source of androgens. In the current state of our knowledge, these are only hypotheses that no argument supports.

The exogenous origin of fetal virilization is, on the other hand, less conjectural. It is indeed certain that the administration to the mother, for a therapeutic purpose, not only androgens, but synthetic progestins, is able to virilize the fetus - and the frequency with which progestins are currently used in the prevention of certain forms of abortion. We must not forget that a hormone can be virilizing for the fetus while it causes no sign of virilism in adults (This is the case, for example, with methyl testosterone).

Here is an example of female pseudo-hermaphroditism, probably due to the mother's testosterone and progesterone injections:

At birth, there is no abnormality, but at the age of one month, the mother notes a clitoral hypertrophy. The growth of the child is normal, the genital abnormality remains unchanged. it is only at the age of 16 months that the child is referred to the service by his doctor for "sex determination". The overall appearance is normal for the chronological age, which confirms the morphologram. In particular, there is no statural advance, nor advance ripening ratios. Bone maturation is also normal, corresponding to the "slow" maturation of 1,5 years (dial method). The examination of the genital area shows the absence of any pubic hair, a relatively short vulvar slit, bordered by pigmented and horizontally folded big lips, coalescing in their 2/3 posterior (picture 3). No mass is perceived during this examination, neither in the labia majora nor in the inguinal canal. At the top of the vulvar cleft, surrounded by it, protrudes the slightly enlarged clitoris; about 1 cm long. Further back is a single perineal orifice. Its opacity objectifies the bladder and a vaginal cavity of normal volume. It is thought to be a female pseudo-hermaphroditism which is confirmed by the female chromatin sex - without adrenal hyperplasia, since there is no sign of hormonal stimulation. The elimination of 17-CS and pregnantriol are indeed normal (before and after ACTH-delay). An exploratory intervention is therefore necessary.

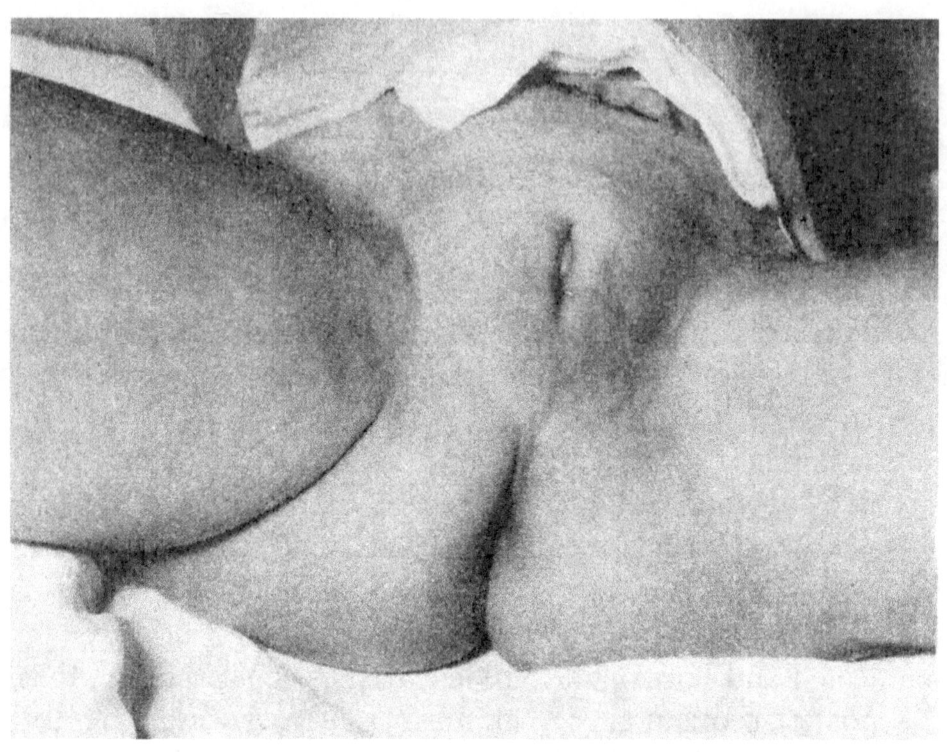

(picture 3) Female pseudo-hermaphroditism due to hormonal injections made to the mother during pregnancy

She shows a

feminine disposition (picture 4) uterus, fallopian tubes and ovaries, whose histological structure will be normal. Only plastic surgical treatment will be necessary to give the clitoris a normal size and enlarge the vulvar cleft.

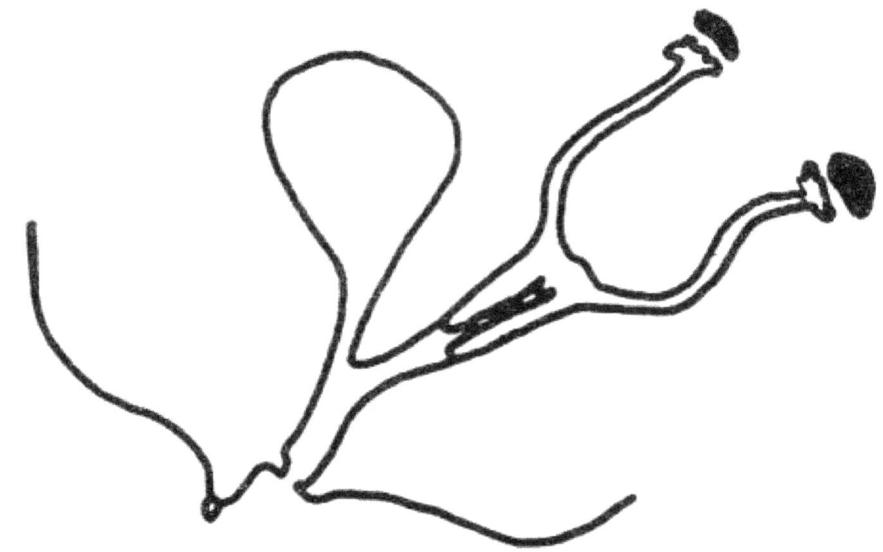

(picture 4) Diagram of the anatomical arrangement of the case of the previous figure

The cause of this partial virilization "in utero" remains, as usual, mysterious. It should be noted, however, that the mother whose pregnancy was unknown then received during the first month 6 injections of testosterone and, for a threat of abortion, 3 injections of progestins during the 4th month.

Therapeutic driving:

In these forms of female pseudo-hermaphroditism, the course of action is simple. By the age of puberty, a local plastic procedure is sufficient to reduce the clitoris to a normal size and sometimes to enlarge the vulvar cleft. The prognosis is also good from a functional point of view: the pubertal evolution is done, of course, according to the normal mode, sexual relations will be established normally, and fertility is possible.

3) The masculine pseudo-hermaphroditism

By definition, the term male pseudo-hermaphroditism refers to a subject with ambiguous external genital morphology, whose chromatin sex is masculine and the gonads are of the testes.

External genital morphology is ambiguous and quite comparable, if not identical, to that described in female pseudo-hermaphroditism, that is to say, realizing the aspect of «hypospadias vulviform», therefore, the external genital configuration should not be relied upon to decide the male or female sex of the child. Of course, in some cases the genital bud, though hypoplastic, clearly evokes a rod, as well as the genital bulges are frankly «bursiform». In any case, there is no orifice at the end of the glans, but a single perineal orifice, located very behind the implantation of the penis. Finally, the gonads are ectopic, perceived or not on the palpation of the inguinal region. Urethrography most often injects a cavity ... vaginal volume and sometimes draws the impression of the cervix. In other cases, there is no visible vaginal cavity which does not prejudge in any way the structure of the internal genital tract. Let's add that the general examination is negative: there is no short stature advance, neither bone advance nor pubic hair, therefore, there is no sign of hormonal stimulation. Hormonal dosages, (in particular 17 CSs) are otherwise normal for the chronological age, at least until puberty.

Surgical exploration shows, in the inguinal or intra-abdominal position, two gonads, whose macroscopic appearance does not allow us to affirm a priori, the male or female nature. Indeed, when the testicles are intra-abdominal, they can be attached to well-individualized tubes, leading or not to a hypoplastic uterus. In other cases, there are no horns, neither uterus, but a deferent-like duct that is lost at the origin of the urethra. In both cases, only the histological examination of a biopsy of the two gonads confirms that these are testicles, with a quasi-normal development of LEYDIG cells, well-differentiated SERTOLI cells, but usually without a recognizable germinal epithelium.

Achieving the diagnosis of male pseudo-hermaphroditism, however, does not solve all the problems, for it remains an extremely grave unknown what the meaning of puberty evolution will be? Indeed, contrary to what one might think since there exist testicles substantially normal histologically, the pubertal development of these children is not always done according to the masculine type, but sometimes according to the feminine type with the feminization of the silhouette and appearance of breasts (Of course, even if there are a vaginal cavity and a uterus there can be no rules since the gonads are testicles).

In practice, it would, therefore, be very important to know in which direction puberty will take place in order to make an early correct decision about the sex of the child. Now, it must be admitted that such prediction is impossible with certainty. The chorionic gonadotropin testicle stimulation test, at a reasonable dose, determines no secretion on an immature testicle, we can not, therefore, using this test try to predict what the testicular secretion will be at the time of puberty. Wilkins insists on the fact, rather singular, that puberty development is all the more likely to be masculine although the internal genital morphology is more feminine. In reality, it is only a probability and we cannot, of the internal genital conformation, draw a definitive argument on the sex to be given to the child. In fact, only plastic surgery, that is to say, can clarify the possibilities offered by the child's reproductive system to reach a functional penis or vagina at the time of puberty, and must decide whether the child will be a boy or a girl - this, of course, in the event that the decision is made early enough so that no psychological considerations will further aggravate the difficulties. It would be a big mistake, on the pretext that the gonads are actually testicles, to want at all costs to make a boy of subjects with a very hypoplastic penis (who will never allow normal sexual intercourse) and who, on the contrary, has a well-developed vaginal cavity.

Therapeutic driving:

It is therefore particularly delicate. If it seems possible to reconstitute a rod that is nearly satisfactory if there is no vaginal cavity, or a very atretic cavity, treat these children as hypospadias - with the addition of a closure of the perineum and, if possible, a lowering of the testicles in general ectopic. (We will take advantage of this lowering to remove the female internal structures). This course of action is obviously the most logical since it concerns male pseudo-hermaphrodites.

When the penis is very aplastic and there is an almost normal vaginal cavity, we will be entitled to practice the necessary interventions for a female morphology as normal as possible.

Of course, one must, in both cases, be ready to practice castration if puberty is not in accordance with the sex assigned to the child. This castration being followed, as the case may be, by the administration of male or female hormones. It must be admitted that the end result is often mediocre.

The following observation illustrates the difficulties encountered in the diagnosis and treatment of these forms of male pseudo-hermaphroditism: the fairly well-developed penis gives the child a distinctly masculine aspect, despite his vulviform hypospadias, however, the internal genital tract is entirely female.

At birth, after a hesitation of a few days, the child is considered a hypospadias boy whose malformation will be corrected later. However, no examination is practiced until the age of 6, when we see it. At this moment, the overall aspect is that of a normal boy for his chronological age, what confirms the morphogram which shows, however, a delay of growth and maturation. Bone maturation is normal (bone age: 6 years, dial method). There is no pubic hair but on palpation of the right inguinal region a mass of soft consistency which cannot be mobilized beyond the lower orifice of the inguinal canal; but there is nothing on the left side. Above all, the external genital morphology is very abnormal of the type «hypospadias vulviform».

The genital bud (picture 5) is quite developed, subtracted by a prolonged brake of a scar, without a meatus at its end, it is visible further back, there is only this single perineal orifice. The scrotum is bifid, undeveloped, surrounding the base of the penis. This very ambiguous aspect allows no conclusion. Complementary exams will show a male chromatin sex and a normal dosages of hormones.

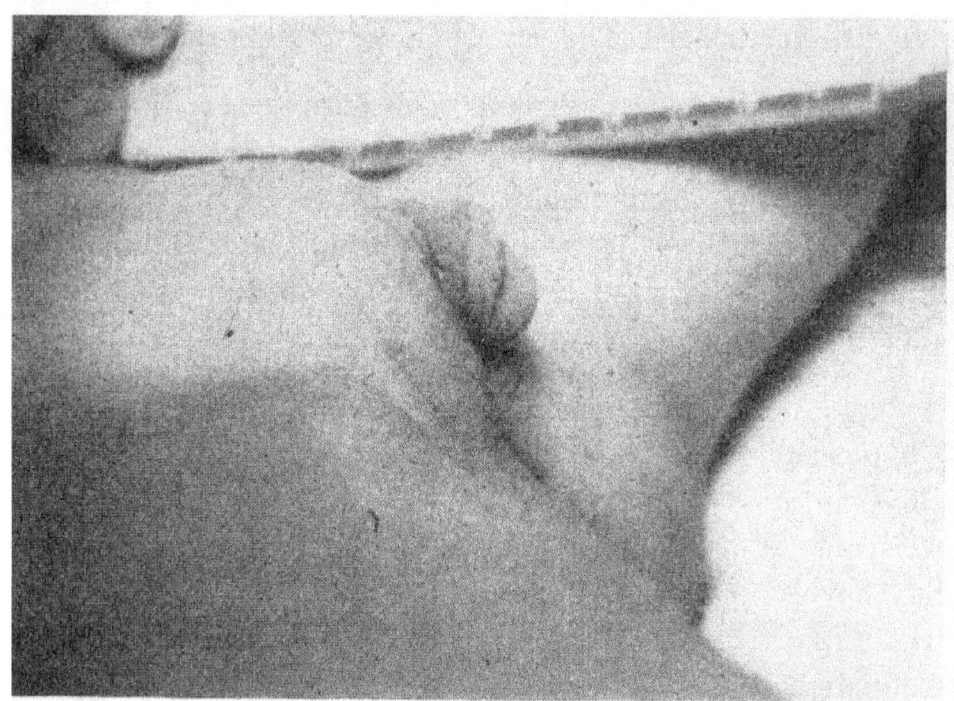

(picture 5) Hypospadias vulviform with fairly well developed penis and bifid scrotum.

The injection of opaque substance through the urethral orifice objective a cylindrical cavity certainly corresponding to a vagina that confirms the exploratory intervention which shows in addition, (picture 6).

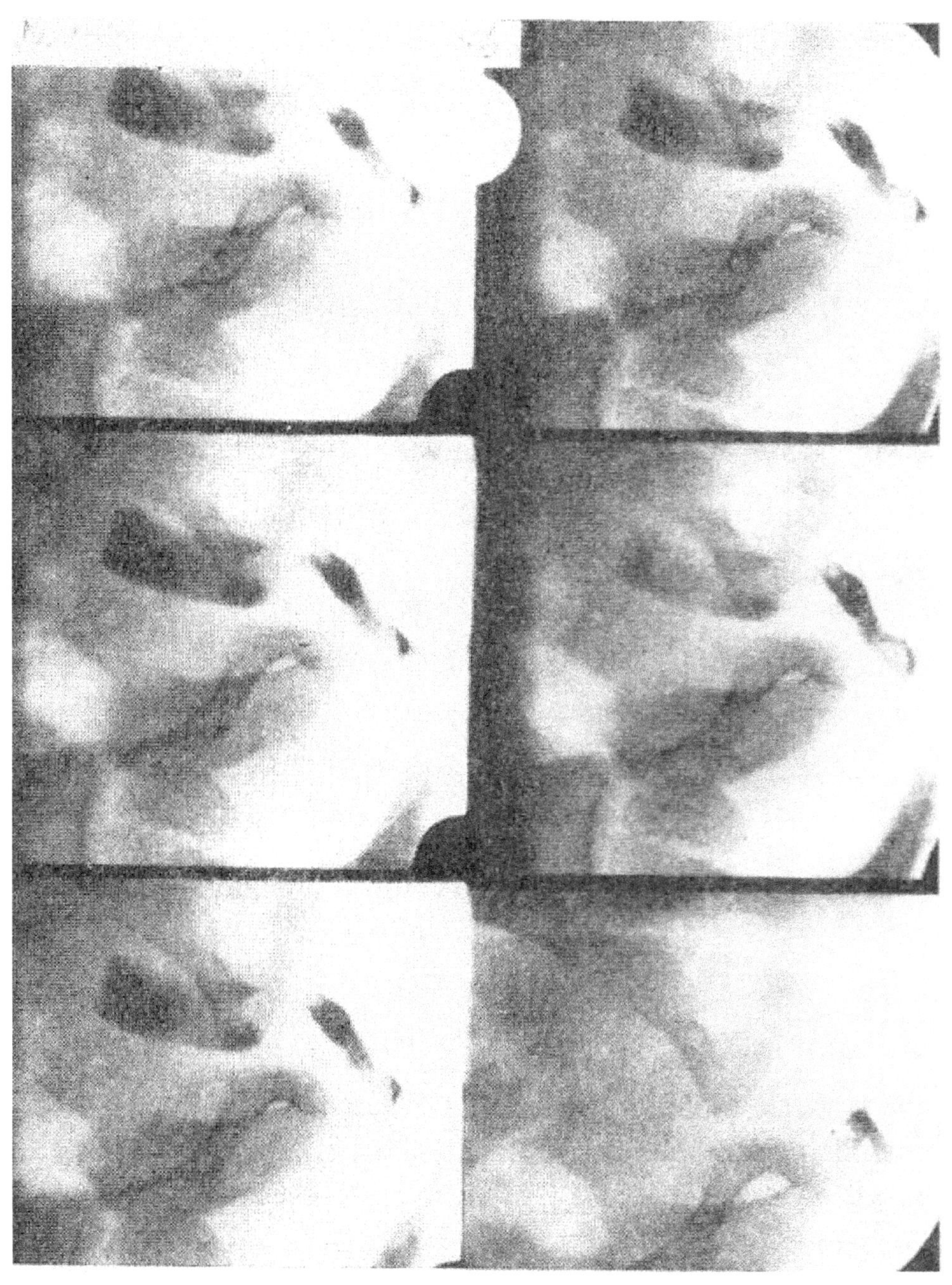

(picture 6) Opacification through the urethral orifice of a well-developed vaginal cavity

back of the bladder, an atrophic uterus, two horns of substantially normal appearance, (picture 7)

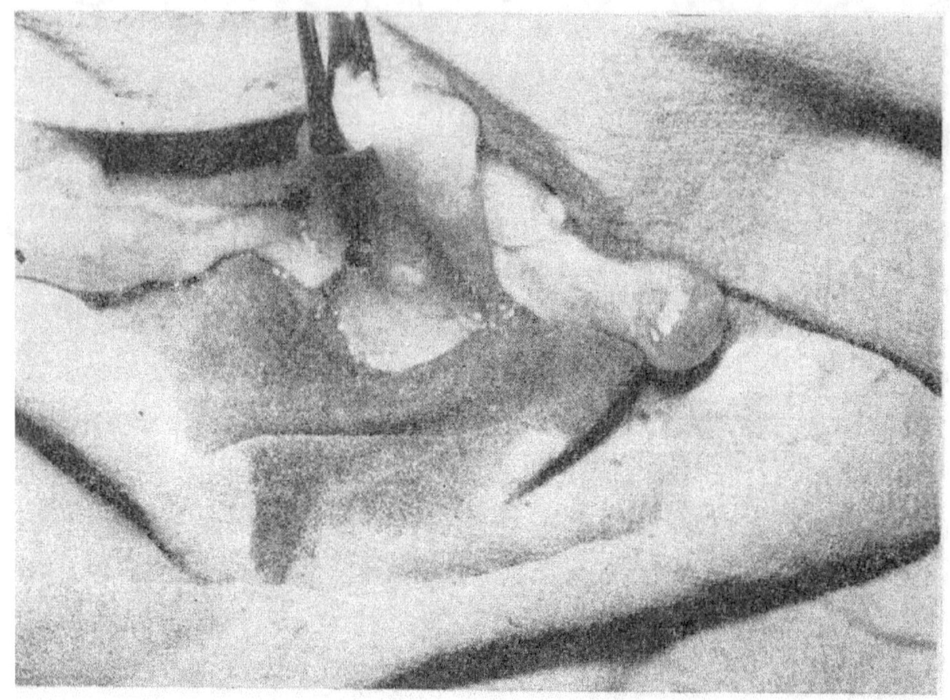

(picture 7) Exploratory intervention uterus tubes and gonads

and two ovoid masses attached to them (picture 8).There is no prostate. Biopsies taken from these two gonad masses show a histological structure of testes (seminiferous tubes well individualized, without hyalinization. The interstitial tissue is poorly developed, but without significant fibrosis).

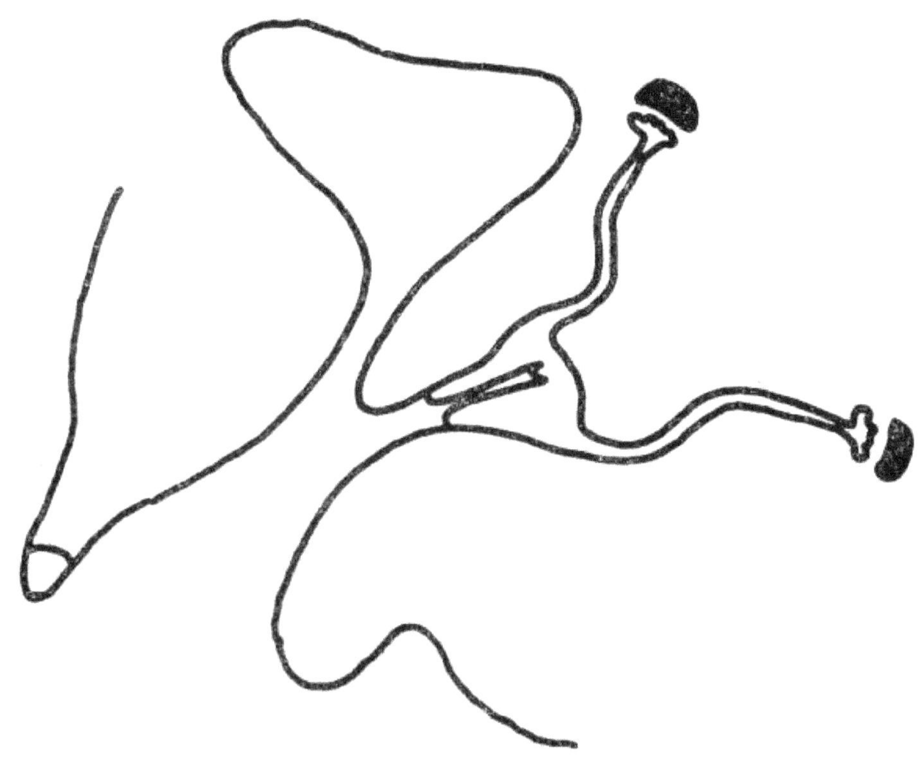

(picture 8) Diagram of the anatomical layout. The gonads are testicles.

It is therefore a pseudo-hermaphroditism male, with an ambiguous external genital morphology with intra-abdominal ectopic testes (the right inguinal mass was formed of cysts, with no trace of testicular tissue), and an internal female genital tract. From a practical point of view, the question is whether, at puberty, the testicles will function as a normal male testis or not. Iterative injections of chorionic gonadotrophin did not cause as expected – there was no testicular secretion. But, the richness in female internal structures is in favor of male puberty.

The child, aged 6, having been raised as a boy until then, it must ,undoubtedly, be kept in this sex, especially that from the purely surgical point of view, it is possible to reconstruct a penile urethra, a subnormal scrotum, and lower the testicles. But of course, if breasts develop at puberty, castration followed by androgen replacement therapy are applied.

Pathogeny:
She must have an explanation why, in subjects whose gonads are testicles, Mullerian regression and external genital differentiation were incomplete. This explanation is provided by the work of Jost. The secretion of the fetal testicle is necessary for the masculinization of the fetus (even of male genetic sex), feminization is on the contrary a passive phenomenon that will occur whenever the fetal testicle is deficient (whatever the genetic sex is). According to the start date and the duration of this deficiency, feminization will be more or less complete (for the notion of critical stages, see image), and is irreversible. This explains the wide variety of abnormalities encountered in ambiguous external genital morphology, assuming, however, that late (between the 3rd and the 5th month) existed an "androgenic" secretion, incomplete, certainly, but sufficient to partially masculinize the perineum. As to why in puberty some cases are female, it must be admitted that it does not appear clearly: here we come to the problem of the "feminizing testicle" which we will discuss later.
4) True Hermaphrodites
True hermaphroditism, that is, the association in a subject with an ambiguous external genital morphology, male and female gonadal tissue is rare. The chromatin sex is masculine or feminine; the genitourinary opacification shows or does not show the presence of a vagina. Only exploratory intervention, therefore, distinguishes these cases from male or female

pseudo-hermaphrodism. In the reported observations of hermaphroditism, these are usually ovotestis, that is to say, the association in each gonad of ovarian and testicular tissue, the genital tract (gonophoric differentiation) presenting the greatest variations. In absolutely exceptional cases, the ovary and its Mullerian apparatus are on one side, the testicle and its differential system are on the other. In any case, it is impossible to predict to what extent the signs of virilization (pilosity) and feminization (breasts) will associate with the moment of puberty. In the same way, no satisfactory explanation has yet been given of gonadogenesis abnormalities which explains the different varieties of true hermaphroditism, that is to say the, persistence during the development of the ambosexual character of the primitive gonad (ovotestis) and even less the development of one side of a male gonad, the other of a female gonad.

Normal external genital aspect: In a second category of facts, the specter of the genitals is masculine or feminine, so there is no apparent ambiguity, we never hesitated about the sex of the child, and yet the study of the different criteria of sexual determination will show that there is some discordance among some of them. But here the consultation is obviously motivated by something other than a doubt about the real sex, and the disorders that lead the child to the doctor's interest about growth or pubertal development. we will first study the cases with female external genital morphology.

**EXTERNAL GENITAL ASPECT IS FEMININE (Table 2).
1) The consultation is motivated by growth disorders**

In some cases, this growth disorder, simple growth retardation or dwarfism, is isolated; but most often this delay is associated with malformations that immediately imposes the diagnosis of Turner Syndrome. The most common of these malformations are the webbed neck, with low hair implantation, ulna valgus and cuirass thorax, in which the complete examination often allows to add aortic coarctation and mental retardation.

The major fact, revealed by the complementary examinations, is the existence of a male chromatin sex (in 80% of cases) whereas the genitourinary opacification objectifies a vagina and the hormonal assays are normal. At the exploration of the small pond or the finding of an infantile uterus, tubes, and under the tubal pavilions, a thin whitish ribbon (genital crestal residue) formed of undifferentiated "sarcomatoid" tissue. These findings correspond to gonadal agenesis, in other cases, it is gonadal dysgenesis, that is to say that the histological examination makes it possible to recognize elements originating from the medulla of the primitive gonad, (rete tubules and Leydig cell-like cell clusters) and sometimes, in the case of female chromatin sex, a rudimentary ovary.

At puberty, there appear only androgenic signs, that is to say a development of pubic hair and labia majora without breast development nor, of course, the appearance of rules. At this time, also the hormonal assays become characteristic, showing an elimination of the 17 CSs, only at a pubertal rate, whereas folliculin is absent and, above all, an abnormal elimination of F S H, greater than 50 mouse units, which signifies the originally gonadal origin of the syndrome.

In complete forms, diagnosis is easy, but it is necessary to think systematically of the possibility of the syndrome of turnérien, Turner syndrome, in the presence of an isolated growth retardation or dwarfism, a mental retardation, and puberty with androgenic signs alone in a child whose external genital morphology is female. In all these cases, the chromatin sex must be studied systematically; if he is masculine, he asserts the diagnosis - the finding of a female sex does not eliminate its absolutely, as we have seen, also note that in front of an infant presenting a predominant edematous syndrome, if not localized, to the lower limbs, and without obvious explanation, it is necessary to study the sex chromatin. if it is masculine, one can affirm the diagnosis of " Bonnevie-Ullrich syndrome", an equivalent of Turner's Syndrome, of which he is only an early manifestation.

Pathogine:

Turner syndromes appear to reproduce in human clinic the embryonic castration experiments of Jost. In fact, everything happens as if the gonads had not developed or disappeared at the very first stage of the differentiation of the genital tract (gonophoric differentiation). Under these conditions, the evolution is, as Jost demonstrated, towards the female type, regardless of the chromatin gender, male or female. But there is no reason, it seems, for the majority (80%) of Turner's syndromes to have a male chromatin sex. Two explanations of this singular predominance have been proposed. For some, it would be a lethal embryo for female embryos, the male embryos being more resistant, hence the greater frequency it is in this sex.

For others, Turner's dysmorphism is a sex-related genetic anomaly; for others, it is an abnormality of the meiosis of the ovum (or spermatozoid). The study of the chromosome balance of the affected individuals and their families will certainly bring information of great interest. Subjects with true Turner syndrome have 45 chromosomes instead of 46 so their chromosome formula would be: AX. So we would understand the high number of "boys", if we admit that the pair XX conditions the presence of the female chromatin corpuscle. In fact, the chromosomal anomaly itself does not seem likely to explain all cases and one comes to wonder what the convenient expression in clinic means of "chromatin sex", "boys" or "girl" when talking about Turner syndrome. Should we not rather consider that these children are of "neutral sex" and that, since their chromosomal formula is neither masculine nor feminine, they develop in the "neutral" sense, meaning, morphologically feminine.

Treatment:
There is not, strictly speaking, a treatment of tumoral syndromes. However one can be led, for a purely psychological purpose, to develop female sexual characteristics by a prolonged administration for several months of estrogen (E.g. Ethinyl estradiol 50% per day) and, in a second time, strive to obtain Pseudo-rules by periodically interrupting estrogen therapy or by doing a cyclic treatment with estrogen and progesterone.

Genital Morphology: Feminine						
Size	Age Bony	Chromatinic sex	Urinary Genital Opacification	Urinary Steroids	Gonads	Observations
Turner's syndrome						
↘	↘	♂ Or ♀	Vagina + Uterus +	N	Agenesis or Dysgenesis	Examined for dwarfism and / or various dystrophies
Male pseudo-hermaphroditism «feminizing testicles»						
N	N	♂	Vagina +	N	Testicles	Examined for «inguinal hernias»
Genital Morphology: male Klinefelter syndrome						
± N	N	♀	Male Urethra	N	Testicles	Examined for «obesity or ectopia»

2) The consultation is motivated by anomalies of pubertal development.

In these cases, the female genital morphology appears not only normal, but also harmonious and, at the usual age of puberty, it starts breast development. But if the breasts gradually acquire a satisfactory volume while the silhouette is feminized, but no other pubertary sign appears: neither genital hair nor menstruation. (Also the study of any primary amenorrhea must systematically include the study of chromatin sex). This dissociation of pubertal signs, especially the contrast between normal breasts and the absence of pubic hair, allows, by the only clinic, to ask almost surely the diagnosis of "Feminizing testicles" (also known as "women's hairless syndrome"), that is, a very particular form of male pseudo-hermaphroditism, Female genital morphology (picture 9).

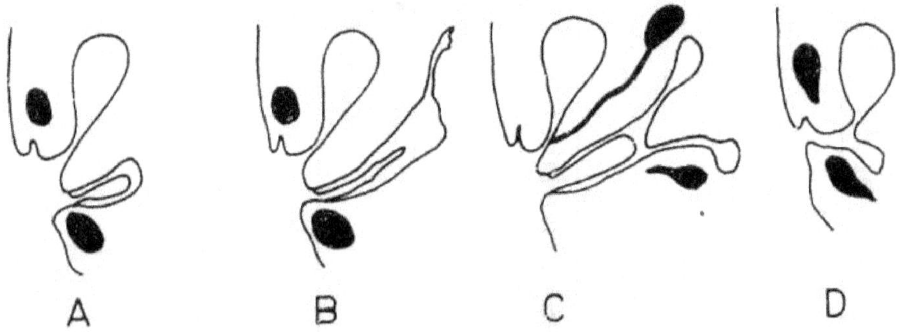

(picture 9) Different anatomical types of male pseudo-hermaphrodism with female external genital morphology (type A most frequent, after WILKINS, modified)

Confirmation is given by the male chromatin sex. The clinical examination can also make it possible to feel the palpation of the inguinal regions, rounded, elastic masses which are actually ectopic gonads, and only the observation of these singular "hernias" could suggest the diagnosis before puberty and lead to the study of the chromatin sex. Sometimes also it will be noted that, if the breast is well developed, the nipple is a little atresic, like the gynecological examination (but it is obviously very difficult) does not perceive uterus, nor annexes. Moreover the injection of opaque substance through the vaginal opening will usually show an atretic cavity, which is sometimes normal.

Finally, at the exploratory laparotomy, the genital tract is non-existent or reduced to a rudimentary deferent. Sometimes there is a sketch of a trunk, and, much more unusually, an atrophic uterus. Before puberty, the histology of the intra-abdominal (or inguinal) gonads does not differ significantly from that of the normal immature testes; after puberty, the interstitial tissue is abundantly developed, the tubes, on the other hand, are generally reduced to the sertolian tissue and an undifferentiated epithelium.

Therapeutic driving:
The morphological aspect of these subjects is absolutely feminine, they have always been raised like files, and it is most often at puberty that they are examined for the first time. In these conditions, no hesitation: they must be kept in the female sex, and even pay the utmost attention to not throwing any trouble in the mind of the child or parents. But should one practice the excision of ectopic testicles?

The only argument in favor of castration is the danger of malignant degeneration. In fact, this danger seems to have been very exaggerated, and does not justify the systematic castration, especially since this is followed by severe menopausal functional disorders. Our tendency would therefore be to leave the testicles in place. An intermediate solution is that proposed by Morris who advises castration once puberty is completed. Of course, an estrogenic replacement treatment is then necessary.

Here is an example we recently observed of this syndrome of «Feminizing testicles» in a 15-year-old girl too, despite breast development, the absence of pubic hair did not seem abnormal. It is the appearance of a right inguinal «mass» which has put on the path of diagnosis.

This girl, now aged 15, was followed in the service since the age of 8 1/2 for a banal obesity. Breast development begins at the age of 13 and continues normally with a nipple that is little salient, no pubic hair appears, but this shift does not worry. It is at nearly 1 years that the child herself notices the presence of a right inguinal «size», and then we evoke the diagnosis of «feminizing testicle» which is affirmed by the male chromatin sex. The vaginal cavity is normal; on the gynecological examination, we do not perceive uterus or appendices. Surgery shows a very hypoplastic uterus. From his right horn is an organ resembling as much an epididymis as a trunk, which joins the inguinal gonad. On the left, the gonad is intra-inguinal, without a differentiated subsidiary organ. On histological examination, these two gonads are testicles with tubes seminiferous features containing spermatogonia and, in the interstitial tissue, there are Leydig cells.

Ultimately, subject to a well-developed vaginal cavity, these male pseudo-hermaphrodites will have a normal female life, but will be sterile and amenorrheic women (Cases reported in adults were only seen the first time at a sterility consultation).

Pathogenesis:

These very singular cases are difficult to understand, especially since their high family incidence must be taken into account, which immediately suggests the idea of a genetically determined anomaly. According to Grumbach and Barr, transmission would be a dominant trait linked to or limited to sex, the mode of action of the pathological gene remains unknown. Whatever the outcome is, no doubt, a partial deficiency of the fetal testicle will exist. The succession of facts would thus be the following during the intrauterine life, the chromosomal sex being masculine (In a case of Danon and Sachs the formula chromosome found was of type AXXY) the gonadogenesis was normal in the direction of the testis. The subsequent testicular deficiency being only partial, it does not persist any significant Muller residues, although the gonophoric differentiation is only incomplete and ambiguous. However, the perineal morphology will be entirely feminine. In addition, feminization must be explained at the time of puberty. But the pubertal testicular secretion is very variable: normal male in our observation and in many others, without an increase in estrogen, besides androgens and estrogens are at female rates - much better, in an observation of Wilkins, estrogens are well at female rates, but androgens (17 CS) are also very high and yet there is no hair system and percutaneous administration or orchids in high doses determines no masculinization. In these circumstances, Wilkins's explanation seems most likely.

This is a syndrome of non receptivity to androgens (Of course, it has been verified that the secreted androgens, measured in the form of 17 CSs were normal, that is to say, led to masculinization when injected into the animal.) where non-receptivity only partially interested in the gonophore, but interesting the urogenital sinus of the intrauterine life (hence the all-female perineal development), the skin and the hair system at the time of puberty. (it should be noted, however, that in about 1/3 of the cases, pubic hair of the female type develops.) Under these conditions, under the influence of pituitary stimuli the testicle works, but only the effects of its estrogenic secretion can be manifested, whether normal or augmented, the «tissue» anomaly also explains the development of aesthetically perfect breasts, but only galactophores. Wilkins, Nelson, and Segal suggested that mothers of infected subjects, during pregnancy, had an anti-testicular antibody; this hypothesis has not, so far, been demonstrated.

It should also be mentioned among the anomalies of the sexual determination with female genital morphology the Congenital Lipoidal Hyperplasia of Adrenal, that we did not show in Table 2 because of its extreme rarity:

We owe it to Prader to describe this anomaly. These are infants whose external genital aspect is absolutely feminine, with a short vagina, dead end, and no uterus. They are seen in the first days or in the first weeks of life for vomiting, diarrhea with a state of collapse expressing acute adrenal insufficiency (as in Debré-Fibiger syndrome); all these children died in the first year of life, the autopsy showing adrenal lipoid hyperplasia and the presence of ectopic testes.

From a practical point of view, it should be noted that in front of a table of "toxicosis" or "pyloric stenosis" in a female infant, if the urinary ionogram shows hypernatruria, if the metabolic disorders are not corrected by the usual treatments, the chromatin sex must be determined; and this one is masculine. This finding asserts the diagnosis and leads to the emergency treatment of adrenal insufficiency.

From a pathogenic point of view, it is certainly a congenital abnormality of adrenal steroidogenesis whose exact stage remains to be specified.

3) EXTERNAL GENITAL ASPECT IS MALE (Table 2)

As in the previous case (female morphology), consultation may be motivated by growth and nutrition disorders, or only later by pubertal abnormalities. The anomalies of growth are variable, delay or the opposite, and especially obesity without particular topographical characters. Isolated or associated with these disorders may be testicular ectopia or mental retardation.

The anomalies of puberty are also variable, it is either pubertal delay, either gynecomastia, or most importantly, for this is the constant sign, dissociated puberty, that is, if the pubic hair and the development of the yard look normal for a teenager, the testicles remain small or atrophic.

In front of these signs, associated or not, before or at puberty, it is necessary to study systematically the chromatin sex that we find feminine which completes to characterize the true Klinefelter syndrome. Hormonal assays will not show anything until puberty. At puberty, the 17 CSs are normal, but the high FSH (greater than 50 US), signing the originally testicular origin of the disease. Indeed, the testicular biopsy will show, on the histological examination, typical alterations of tubular sclerohyalinosis with very a reduced or absent spermatogenesis and a substantially normal development of Leydjg cells. Very importantly, it was believed that these old testicular lesions were scarring witnesses fetal gonadogenesis disorders. However, since we know how to make the diagnosis before puberty thanks to the systematic study of chromatin sex, it was found that the histological appearance of the testicle may still be normal and we studied four such observations. (including one with ambiguous morphology). Therefore, sclerohyalinosis is not the fundamental phenomenon, it can only develop at puberty (under the influence of the FSH) and one could, perhaps, avoid it.

Treatment:
Actually, this is, for the moment only a hypothesis, and no effective treatment can yet be proposed. In classic forms recognized in adolescence, there is no treatment, virility is normal (normal androgenic secretion) and one can not, of course, at this stage, hope to influence definitive sclerosing lesions of the germ line. The sexual behavior of these subjects is therefore normal, but they will be sterile.

Pathogenesis:
There is very likely a gene tare causing true Klineflter syndrome. The chromosome balance is abnormal, of formula AXXY, so with a total of 47 chromosomes instead of 46 (the presence of XX would explain, as we said before, the female chromatin sex). In fact, this chromosomal anomaly does not make it possible to understand the familial cases of Klineflter such as those reported by Reifenstein, moreover, the very mechanism of gonadal inversion remains unknown. Witschi

invoked the absence of gonadal colonization, but this hypothesis seems to be invalidated by observations that signal spermatogenesis. Similarly, the absence of "cortecine" or a congenital metabolic abnormality of the inducers of the gonad are so far only working hypotheses.

We still have to report very rare cases (and not listed for this reason in Table II) congenital adrenal hyperplasia in fully virilized girls, so that the external genital morphology is absolutely masculine, although it is female pseudo hermaphroditism. In the neonatal period, they can only be recognized if they appear in the form of Debre-Fibiger syndrome, otherwise the diagnosis can be made only when the sexual hair and the spring advance appear by the discovery of a female chromatin sex. These forms of hyperplasia are the only ones where breeding sex must be left masculine.

In this lesson, we have presented the main data on sexual ambiguities (on the one hand, Gonadic dysgenesis, including Klinefelter's Turner syndromes and True Hermaphroditism; on the other hand, pseudo-Hermaphrodism masculine and feminine). We must insist on the importance of the psychological problems posed by all these cases, such importance that from a certain age the possibilities of somatic treatment are subordinated to psychological data. We can not undertake here the detailed study, but we want to insist strongly on the absolute necessity of an early decision. Indeed, the psychology of the child is very early oriented towards masculinity or femininity. Without going so far as to affirm the psychic sexualization of the young infant, the care of the entourage,
the different way in which we raise a boy and a girlthat at the age of 2 years, the «psychological sex» is already so fixed that

it is very difficult and risky to undertake a «sex change». Wilkins, Money, Hampson formally discourage any attempt of this kind, under penalty of disasters. It is therefore essential to arrive as soon as possible, from the first months, to a precise diagnosis of the sex in which the child will have to be raised, because we can then make a decision that takes into account only real anatomical and functional possibilities. This is the essential notion. In all cases, a simple examination is possible from birth by the study of chromatin sex. While waiting for the other complementary examinations, it is advisable that the child be declared according to his chromatin sex.

Unfortunately, and our observations are examples, children are too often examined late that sometimes they are not examined before 17. What attitude should be adopted then, in other words - to the extent that anatomy gives the possibility - can one still, from the psychological point of view, propose a sex change? Most writers do not think so, a change may only be possible much later, to adolescence or adulthood, if the subject himself solicits it. The discussion must in fact be repeated in each particular case because it poses problems not only of technique, but also of medical ethics.

We will conclude by saying that thanks to an early examination, rigorous and systematic of any suspicious case, these subjects will be given the maximum chance of leading a somewhat normal life (adrenal hyperplasia), or at least the most acceptable life possible (Pseudo-Hermaphrodism).

Bibliographic indications

JONES (H.W.) and Scott (W.W) Hermaphroditism, Genital anomalies, and related endocrine. The Williams and Wilkins ed. Baltimore, 1958.

WILKINS (L). The diagnosis and treatment of endocrine disorders in childhood and adolescence. C.S. Thomas, ed. Springfield, Illinois, 1985. (2° edition).

SEBAOUN-ZUCMAN (M). Les états intersexués d'origine gonadique. These Paris, 1958.

Actualités Pédiatriques, Troisième Série, Search by Pierre CANLORBE Paris, 1961.